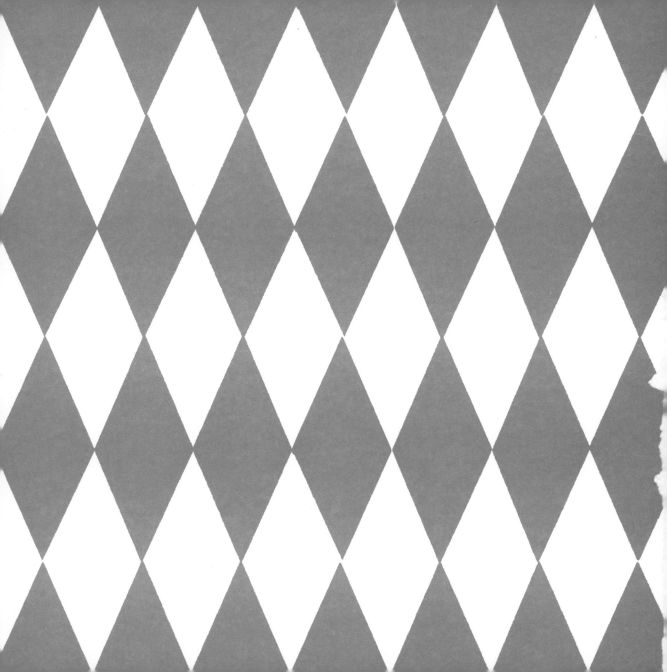

DAD*ICATED*

MADE FOR YOU BY...

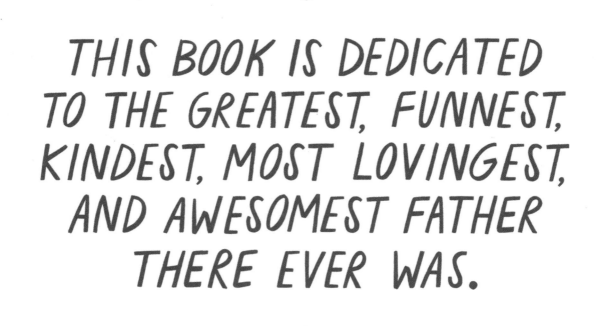

THIS BOOK IS DEDICATED TO THE GREATEST, FUNNEST, KINDEST, MOST LOVINGEST, AND AWESOMEST FATHER THERE EVER WAS.

THIS BOOK IS DEDICATED TO YOU,

_____.

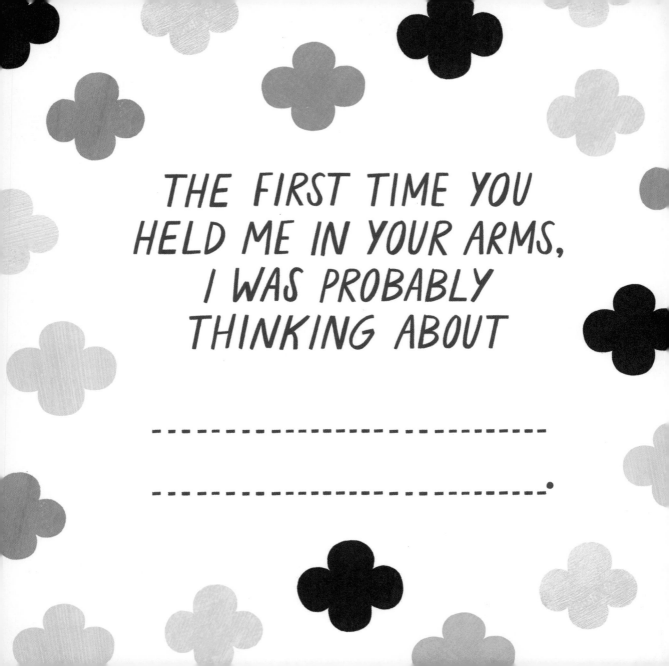

THE FIRST TIME YOU HELD ME IN YOUR ARMS, I WAS PROBABLY THINKING ABOUT

---.

OTHER DADS ARE

· ·

AND

· .

BUT YOU'RE

· ·

AND NEVER

!

· ·

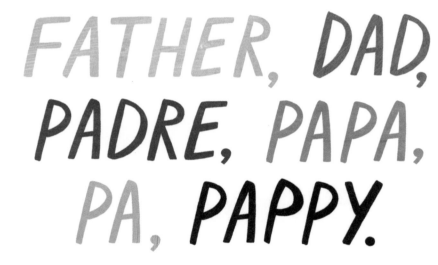

FATHER, DAD, PADRE, PAPA, PA, PAPPY.

BUT TO ME YOU'LL ALWAYS BE

_____.

I'VE NEVER UNDERSTOOD
HOW YOU MAKE

· ·

· ·

· ·

LOOK SO DARN EASY,
BUT YOU DO.

ONE OF MY MOST FAVORITE MEMORIES OF YOU AND ME FROM WHEN I WAS A KID IS THIS ONE:

REMEMBER THAT
TIME I SAID

....

....

....?

I'M SO SORRY!
I DIDN'T MEAN IT!

BUT WHEN I SAY

_____

_____

_____

NOW, I DEFINITELY
MEAN EVERY WORD.

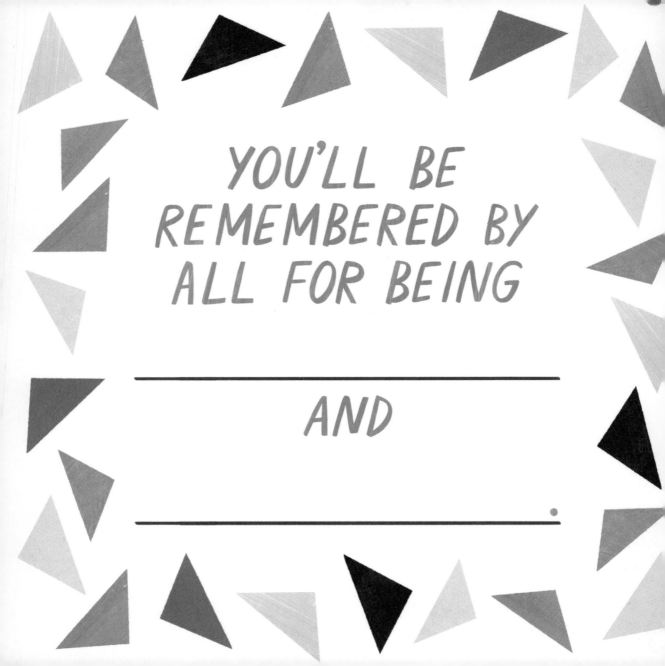

YOU'LL BE
REMEMBERED BY
ALL FOR BEING

_____

AND

_____

EVERY TIME I HEAR

....

OR SEE

....,

I ALWAYS THINK
OF YOU.

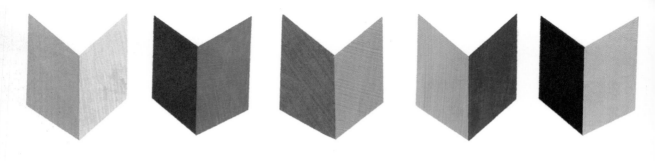

IF I WERE TO WRITE A BEST-SELLING BOOK ABOUT YOU, IT WOULD BE TITLED

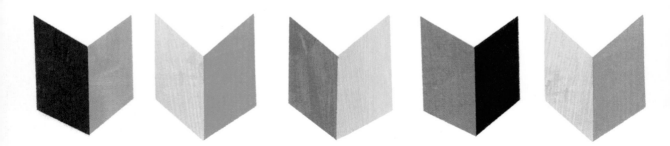

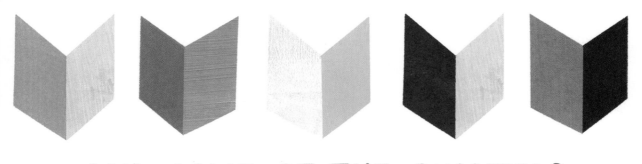

AND SOME OF THE CHAPTERS
WOULD BE CALLED

-----------------------------,

-----------------------------,

AND

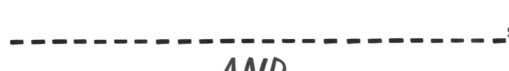

-----------------------------.

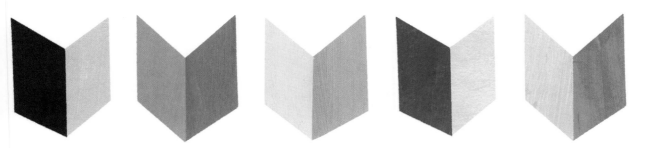

DAD,

I LOVE YOU MORE THAN

· ·

AND · .

AND WAY MORE THAN

· ,

IF YOU CAN BELIEVE IT!

ONE OF MY MOST FAVORITE THINGS TO DO WITH YOU IS

_____

_____ .

I KNOW YOU LOVE ME
FOR SURE BECAUSE
OF THE WAY YOU

....

....

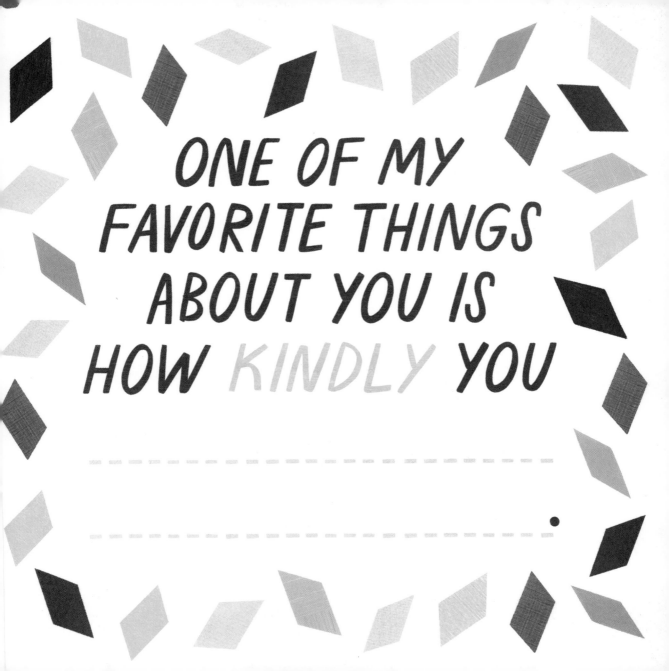

ONE OF MY
FAVORITE THINGS
ABOUT YOU IS
HOW KINDLY YOU

---------------------------------- .

YOU'RE MY GO-TO GUY EVERY TIME I

I DON'T THINK I'D KNOW HOW TO DO IT WITHOUT YOU.

REMEMBER THAT
TIME YOU AND I

------------------------- ?

I LOVED THAT DAY!

YOU ARE PRETTY MUCH
GOOD AT EVERYTHING!
YOU CAN

WITHOUT EFFORT,
YOU CAN PROBABLY

WITH YOUR EYES CLOSED...

AND YOU CAN EVEN

_____ .

BUT I HAVE TO SAY,
YOU'RE NOT THE BEST AT

_____ .

BUT ME NEITHER!

YOU MAY BE TIRED, STRESSED, WORN OUT, AND EVEN

————— ————— ————— ————— ————— ————— ————— ————— ————— —————,

BUT YOU NEVER FAIL TO

————— ————— ————— ————— ————— ————— ————— ————— ————— —————.

I ADMIRE YOU FOR THIS SO MUCH.

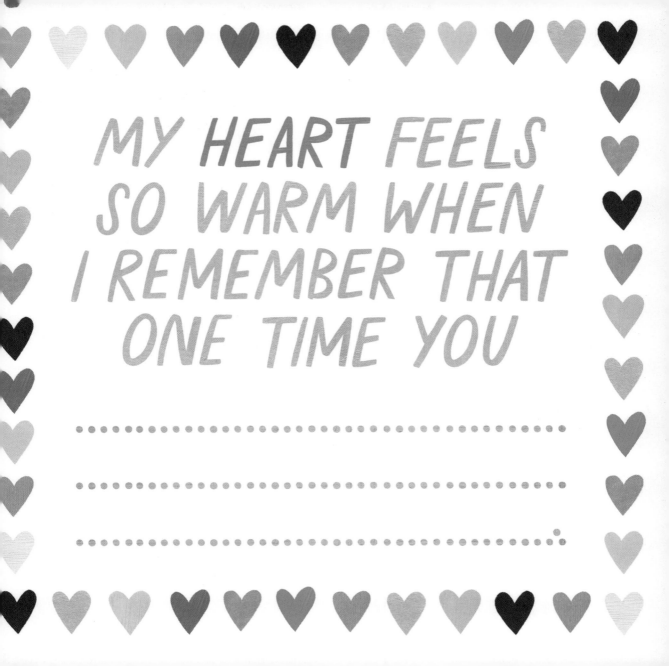

MY HEART FEELS
SO WARM WHEN
I REMEMBER THAT
ONE TIME YOU

....

....

....

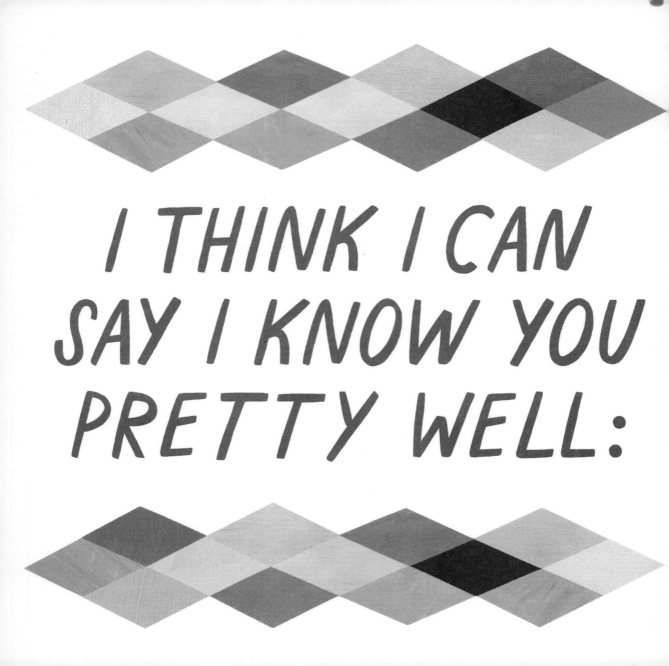

I THINK I CAN SAY I KNOW YOU PRETTY WELL:

YOU WOULD NEVER EVER EAT

_____,

BUT _____

IS ONE OF YOUR FAVORITE SNACKS.

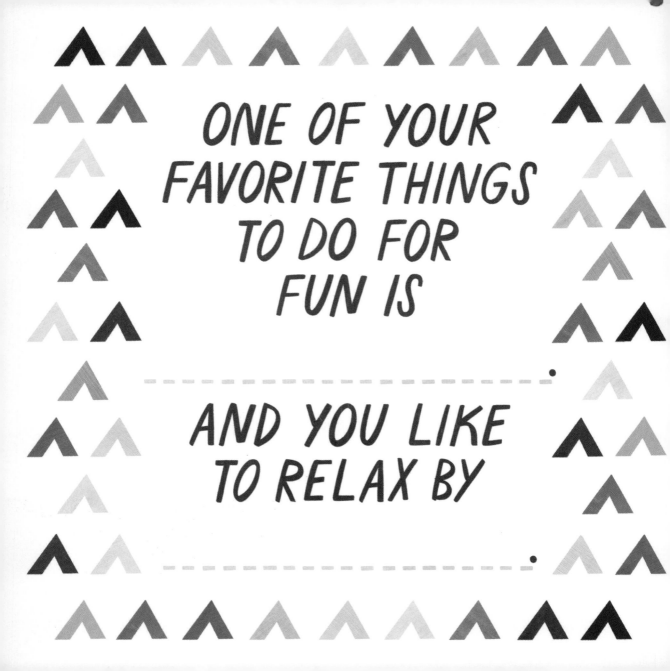

ONE OF YOUR
FAVORITE THINGS
TO DO FOR
FUN IS

------------------------------ .

AND YOU LIKE
TO RELAX BY

------------------------------ .

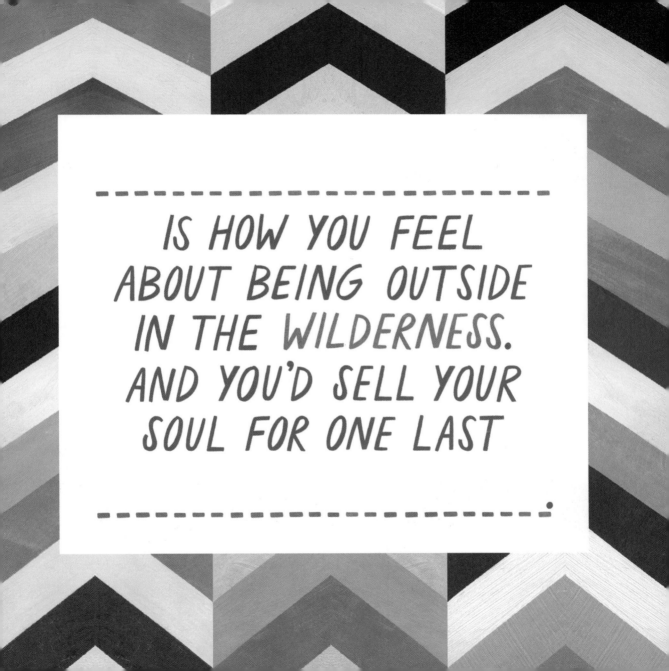

IS HOW YOU FEEL
ABOUT BEING OUTSIDE
IN THE WILDERNESS.
AND YOU'D SELL YOUR
SOUL FOR ONE LAST

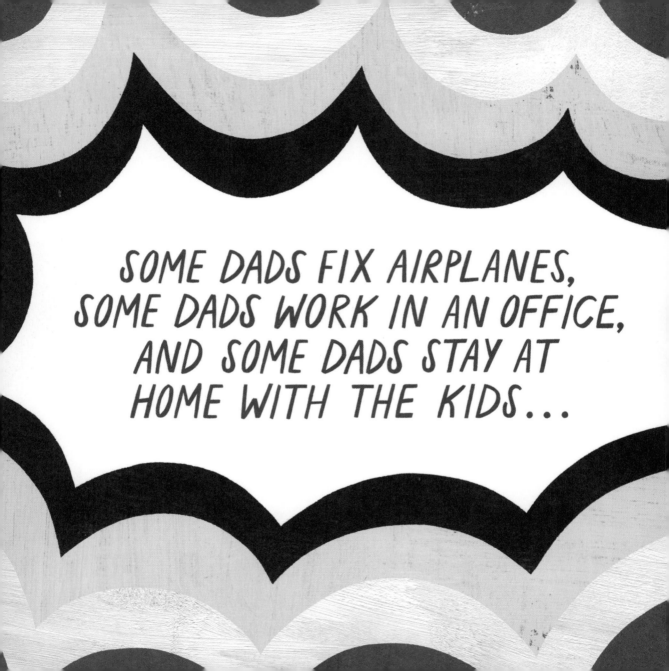

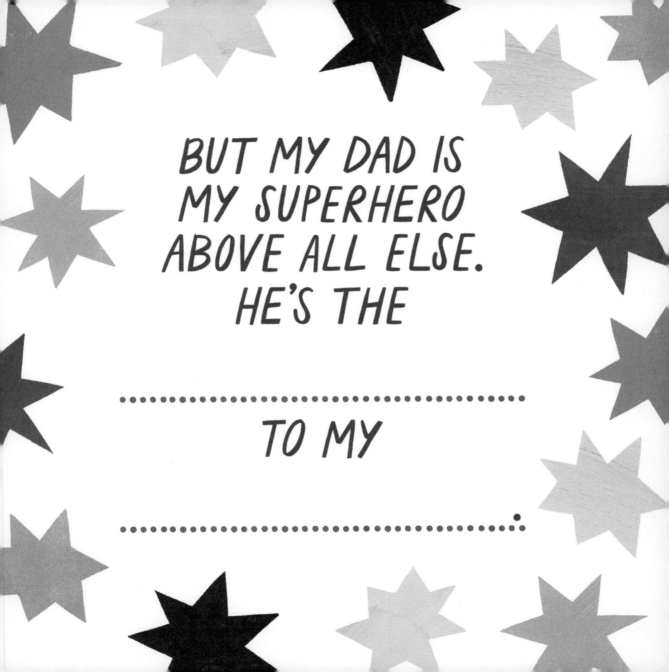

BUT MY DAD IS
MY SUPERHERO
ABOVE ALL ELSE.
HE'S THE

....

TO MY

....

DESPITE IT BEING MIDNIGHT, I'D STILL CALL YOU IF I NEEDED

I MAY HAVE OUTGROWN

AND_____,
BUT I'LL NEVER OUTGROW
MY NEED FOR YOUR

------------------------------------.

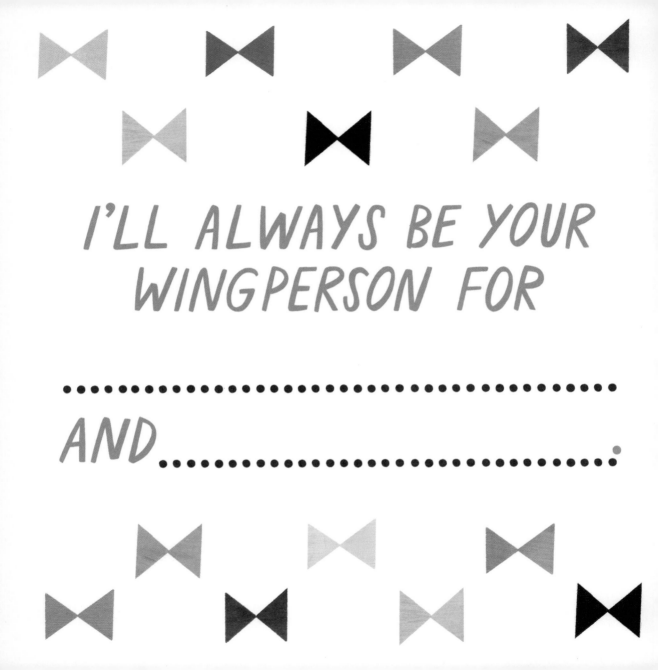

I'LL ALWAYS BE YOUR
WINGPERSON FOR

....

AND..

DAD,

YOU'RE THE ONLY PERSON
IN THE WHOLE WORLD
I'D EVER WANT TO GO

WITH.

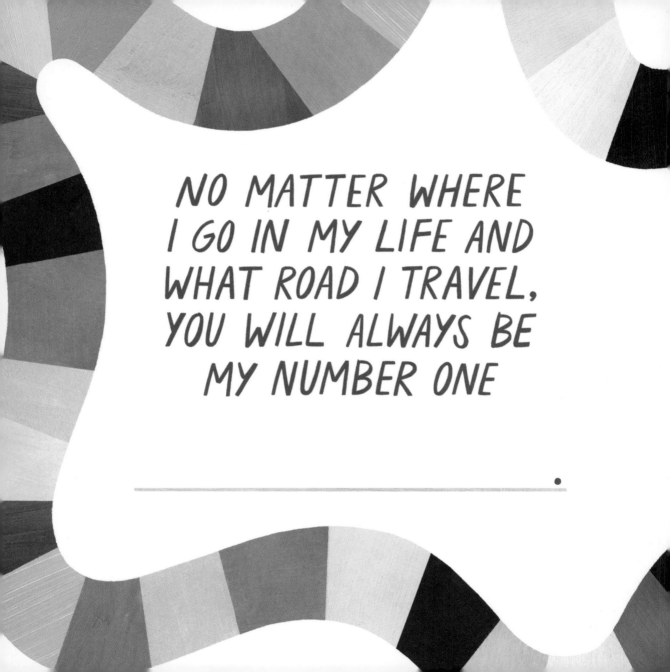

WHETHER IT'S BACKPACKING
TRIPS TO THE TOP OF THE WORLD,
MOVIE NIGHT ADVENTURES WITH
POPCORN AND CANDY, OR

_____ ,

I ALWAYS CHERISH MY TIME
WITH YOU.

FATHER /ˈfäTHər/

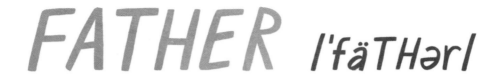

1 A PERSON WHO IS
.... BEYOND
.............................:

2 A LOVING ....
WITH A BRAVE ....:

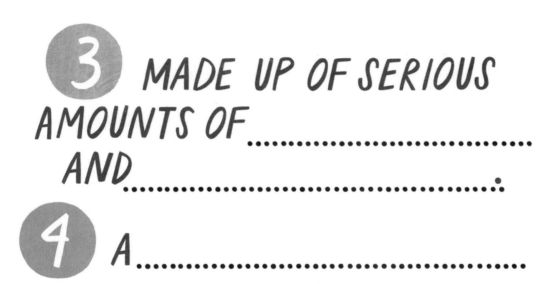

3 MADE UP OF SERIOUS AMOUNTS OF.. AND...:

4 A... LIKE NO OTHER.

WE CAN BE SO DIFFERENT
AT TIMES, BUT I'M
STILL A CHIP OFF THE
OLD BLOCK BECAUSE

------------------------------ .

ALSO, WE'RE PRACTICALLY IDENTICAL IN THE WAY WE

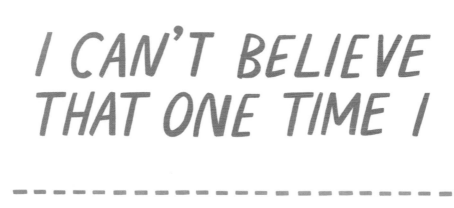

I CAN'T BELIEVE
THAT ONE TIME I

------------------------------.

YOU DEFINITELY
WEREN'T HAPPY
ABOUT IT...

BUT YOU STILL

. . . .

ME ANYWAY.
BECAUSE YOU'RE JUST SO
WONDERFUL LIKE THAT.
AND I NEVER

. . . .

AGAIN!

EVERY TIME I NEED
TO KNOW HOW TO

__ __ __ __ __ __ __ __ __ __

__ __ __ __ __ __ __ __ __ __ ,

I CALL YOU!

REMEMBER THAT

· ·

· ·

YOU GAVE ME WHEN I WAS YOUNGER? I STILL HAVE IT!

I HAD NEVER TRIED

BEFORE.
BUT WITH YOU,
I TRIED IT AND
ABSOLUTELY
IT.

ONE OF MY MOST FAVORITE
THINGS YOU COOK IS

_____.

I HOPE THAT I CAN
LEARN TO MAKE THIS
JUST AS GOOD AS YOU DO!

I LAUGH EVERY
SINGLE TIME
I THINK ABOUT
THAT TIME WE

....
....
....!

IT'S A TOSS-UP.
I CAN'T DECIDE IF
YOU ARE MORE

_ _

OR MORE

_ .

_ _

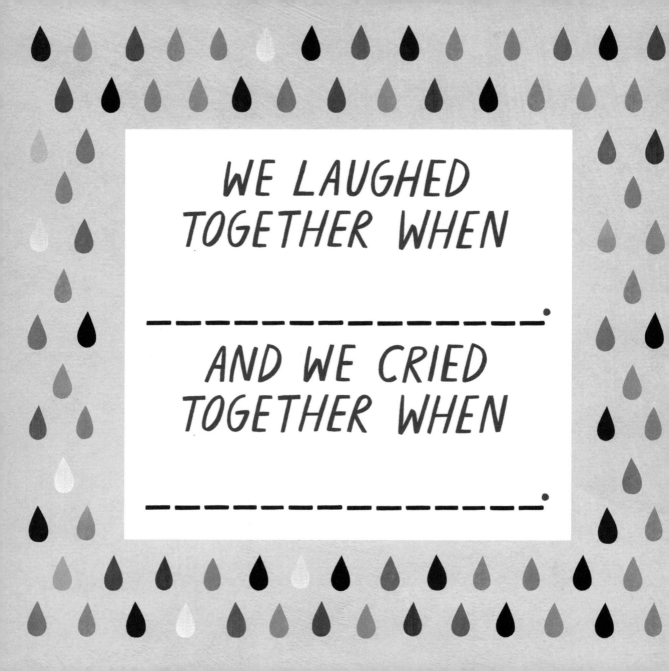

WE LAUGHED
TOGETHER WHEN

————————————————·

AND WE CRIED
TOGETHER WHEN

————————————————·

I REALLY THINK
THAT ALL DADS ARE

IN DISGUISE.

YOU ARE WITHOUT A DOUBT MY ABSOLUTE FAVORITE PERSON TO _____ WITH.

TO THE WORLD,
YOU MAY JUST BE A DAD.
BUT TO ME, YOU ARE

....

AND YOU ARE

....

ABOVE ALL ELSE.

I KNOW THAT YOU LOVE ME FOR

------- -- -- -- --- -- -- -- -- -- --- -- -- -- -- -- --- -- --

-- -- --- -- -- -- -- -- --- -- -- -- -- -- --- -- -- -- -- --

AND ACCEPT ME FOR

------- -- -- -- --- -- -- -- -- -- --- -- -- -- -- -- --- -- --

-- -- --- -- -- -- -- -- --- -- -- -- -- -- --- -- -- -- -- -- .

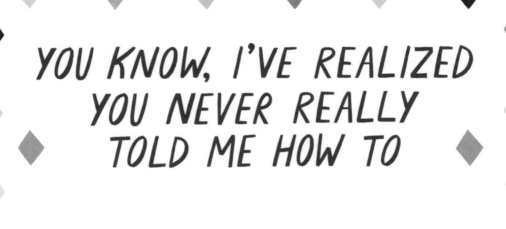

YOU KNOW, I'VE REALIZED
YOU NEVER REALLY
TOLD ME HOW TO

_____.

BUT I LEARNED THIS
BY WATCHING YOU DO IT.

SOME DADS ARE FROM
SMALL TOWNS LIKE
MILLEDGEVILLE, GEORGIA.

AND SOME DADS ARE
FROM BIG CITIES
LIKE NEW YORK CITY.

BUT NO MATTER WHERE
DADS COME FROM,
THEY ALL SEEM TO SHARE
THIS ONE SPECIAL TRAIT:

_ .

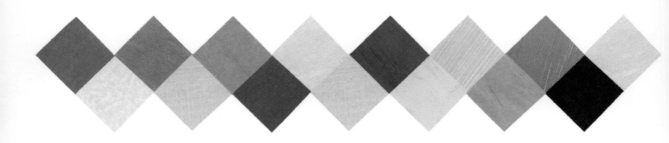

YOU HAVE 1/4 PATIENCE,
1/2 UNDERSTANDING,
1/4 WIT, AND AN ENTIRE
BEING FULL OF

_____.

....

....

HAS BEEN ONE OF THE
GREATEST THINGS
I'VE LEARNED FROM YOU.
I TRY TO EMULATE
THIS EVERY DAY.

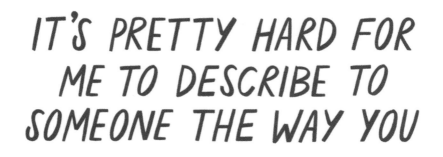

IT'S PRETTY HARD FOR
ME TO DESCRIBE TO
SOMEONE THE WAY YOU

_____

_____

_____ .

BUT IT'S ONE OF MY
FAVORITE THINGS
ABOUT YOU.

IF YOU AND I WERE THROWN IN JAIL FOR A NIGHT, IT WAS PROBABLY BECAUSE

....

....:

LET'S PLAN THE ULTIMATE
MOVIE NIGHT TOGETHER!
FOR THE MOVIE GENRE,
WE'D OBVIOUSLY CHOOSE A
_____ MOVIE.

AND WE'D WATCH IT AT
_____ HOUSE.

AND WE'D MAKE SURE
TO HAVE LOADS OF

_____.

SNACKS? WE'D
DEFINITELY HAVE

_____

AND_____.

AND I DON'T KNOW
ABOUT YOU, BUT
I'D BE DRINKING A
NICE TALL GLASS OF

_____.

DADS SEEM TO ALWAYS BE SO GOOD AT MAKING THEIR CHILDREN FEEL SAFE AND PROTECTED.

REMEMBER THAT ONE TIME

------------------------------ ?

I WAS TERRIFIED! BUT
YOU HELPED ME TO FEEL

BY

------------------------------ .

YOU'RE THE FUNNIEST
GUY I KNOW!
NO REALLY, YOU ALWAYS
SEEM TO MAKE EVERYONE

WHEN YOU TELL YOUR
JOKES OR STORIES.

ONE OF MY FAVORITE FUNNY STORIES YOU TELL IS THIS ONE:

_____

_____

_____

_____.

WHEN I WAS A KID,
YOU TOLD ME

------------------------------ .

AND TO THIS DAY,
I STILL THINK

------------------------------ .

I MAY NOT SAY IT AS OFTEN AS I SHOULD, BUT DAD, I

....

I ....

A WHOLE DANG LOT!

ONE OF THE
CRAZIEST THINGS
I'VE EVER SEEN
YOU DO WAS

_____

_____

_____

AND ONE OF THE KINDEST THINGS I'VE EVER SEEN YOU DO WAS

· ·

· ·

· ·

IT DOESN'T SEEM TO MATTER HOW CRAZY LIFE CAN GET, BECAUSE YOU'RE ALWAYS THERE TO _____

_____

AND _____ .

AND ESPECIALLY TO _____ !

_____

SOMETHING YOU DID
WITH ME AS A KID
THAT I THINK EVERY
DAD SHOULD DO WITH
THEIR LITTLE ONE IS

....

....

I DON'T KNOW ABOUT ANYONE ELSE, BUT I FEEL LIKE ALL DADS HAVE THESE CERTAIN SAYINGS. FOR INSTANCE, SOME DADS SAY, "DON'T MAKE ME PULL THIS CAR OVER!" AND SOME DADS SAY, "MONEY DOESN'T GROW ON TREES!"

YOU CERTAINLY HAVE YOUR OWN SAYINGS AS WELL! THESE ARE SOME OF MY FAVORITES:

YOU ARE SO MANY THINGS ALL AT ONCE. BUT YOU ARE THESE ABOVE ALL!

FANTASTICALLY _____
    AND _____.

A _____ SOUL WITH A KIND _____.

THE ONLY PERSON I TRUST BEYOND
    MEASURE TO _____.

HILARIOUSLY _____ WHEN YOU
    TRY TO _____.

ENCOURAGING AND _____
    WHEN I NEED IT THE MOST.

REASSURING. YOU ALWAYS MAKE ME FEEL
    _____ WHEN I AM

DOWN IN THE DUMPS.

IF I DIDN'T HAVE YOU AS THE **MOST WONDERFUL** DAD THAT I DO, I'D CHOOSE YOU AS A

....

BECAUSE I CAN'T IMAGINE
_____ WITHOUT
YOU IN IT. YOU GAVE ME ONE
OF THE GREATEST GIFTS I'VE
EVER RECEIVED—YOU GAVE ME
_____. AND I'M
A MUCH BETTER PERSON TODAY
BECAUSE OF _____.
THANK YOU, DAD, FOR BEING
MY _____.

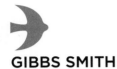

GIBBS SMITH
TO ENRICH AND INSPIRE HUMANKIND

25 24 23 22 21   5 4 3 2 1

Written by Kenzie Lynne, © 2021 Gibbs Smith

Illustrated by Melanie Mikecz, © 2021 Melanie Mikecz

Published by
Gibbs Smith
P.O. Box 667
Layton, Utah 84041

1.800.835.4993 orders
www.gibbs-smith.com

Designed by Melanie Mikecz

Printed and bound in China
Gibbs Smith books are printed on either recycled, 100% post-
consumer waste, FSC-certified papers or on paper produced
from sustainable PEFC-certified forest/controlled wood source.
Learn more at www.pefc.org.

ISBN: 978-1-4236-5719-4

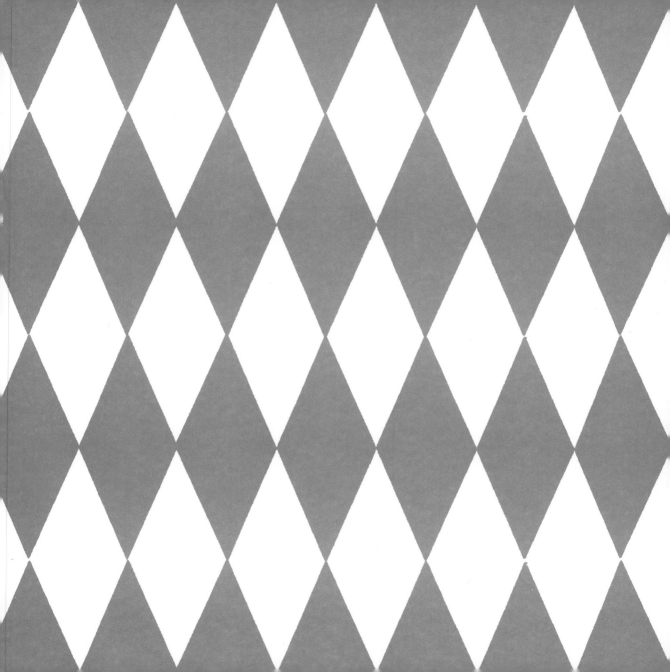

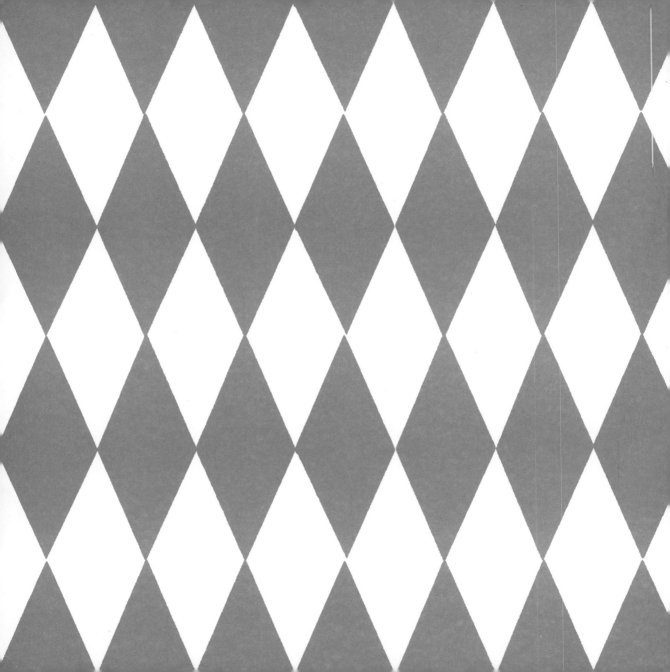